This book belongs to:

_____

Kids On Screen

By: Neeti Kohli, M.D.

Kids on Screen

To order additional copies of this book, contact:

Awareness Books for Children
P.O. Box 2495
Edmond, Oklahoma 73083-2495

Phone: 1-405-330-8888
Fax: 1-405-330-8880

Website: www.awarenessbooksforchildren.org

THANK YOU

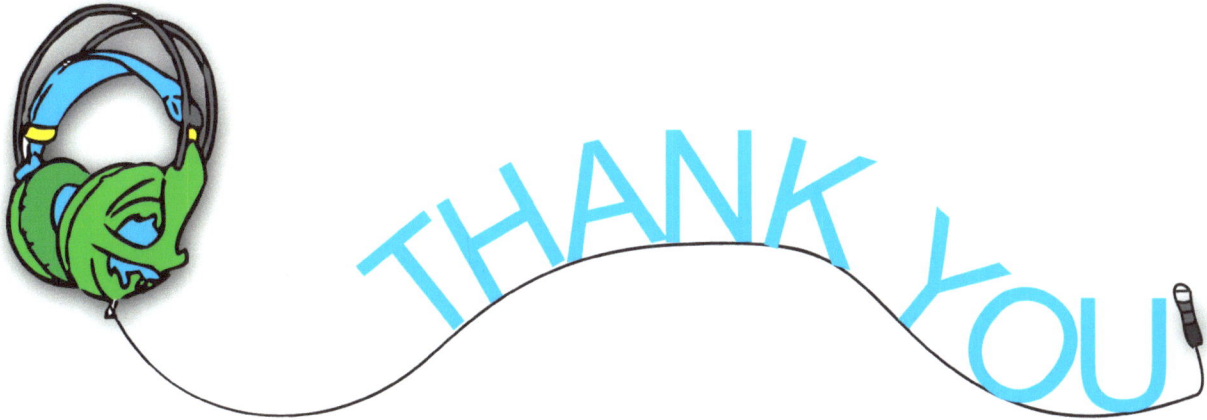

My special thanks to:

My husband Vivek and
my children Uday & Supriya

Xlibris Publication

Kristi Kenney

Randy Anderson

Wayne Stein

Family & Friends

A note to parents

Children have started to overuse their access to electronics that possess screens. Televisions, computers, cell phones, video games, and other portable devices have become very common these days. Many scientific studies have documented some bad effects of these devices.

As technology is advancing very rapidly, it is important to be proficient in using these devices. However, they come with a load of harmful effects that may not be so obvious.

Parents as well as students aren't realizing the potential harm that screens may cause. One should always be prepared to handle a problem before it reaches an extreme level. Otherwise, it will be too late to correct it.

This book was written to raise awareness in our children, so that they can differentiate between the good and bad effects of the screen from a very early age. It is based on the recommendations by the American Academy of Pediatrics and is written with the hope to bring about a positive change in our society. Enjoy reading this book with your kids!

Best Wishes,
Neeti Kohli, M.D.

Kids On Screen

All of us have televisions, computers, video games, cell phones, and other electronics at home and school.

We should know how to use these devices for our best benefit.

A lot of advantages come from working with them.

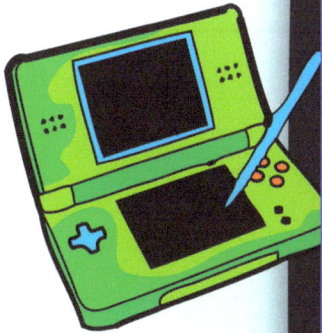

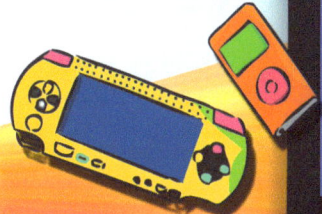

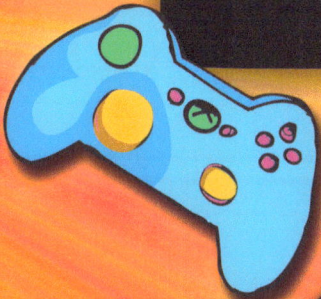

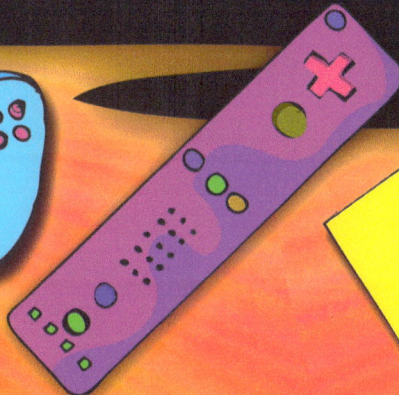

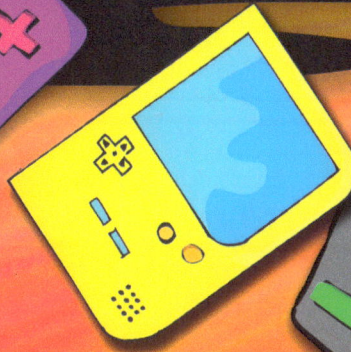

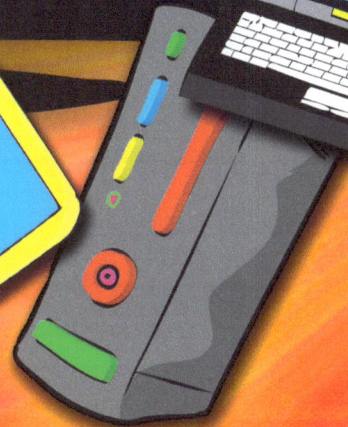

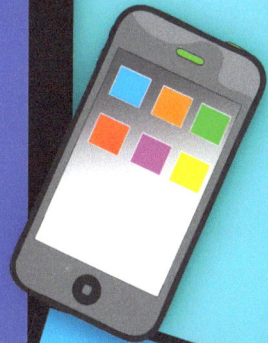

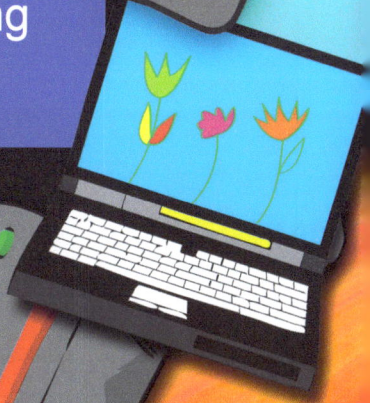

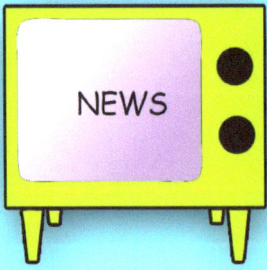

NEWS

TELEVISIONS

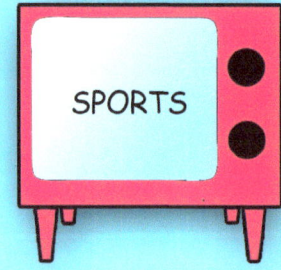

SPORTS

So many good shows
can be seen
as we travel around the world
while relaxing on a seat.

Entertainment

Live Broadcast

Television teaches us good things
that we need to know.
It tells us about news
to make our minds grow.

Sing Along

Talent Show

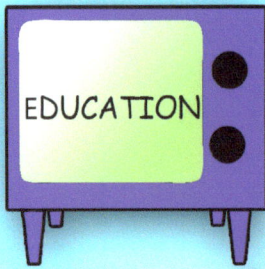

EDUCATION

If the weather is bad,
it sounds an alarm,
so that it can save us
from any kind of harm.

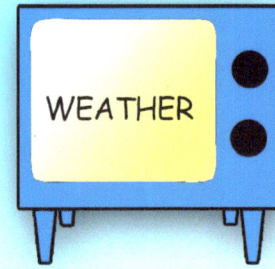

WEATHER

It makes us laugh,
sing and dance.
We all begin to see
our moods enhance.

Dance

Exercise

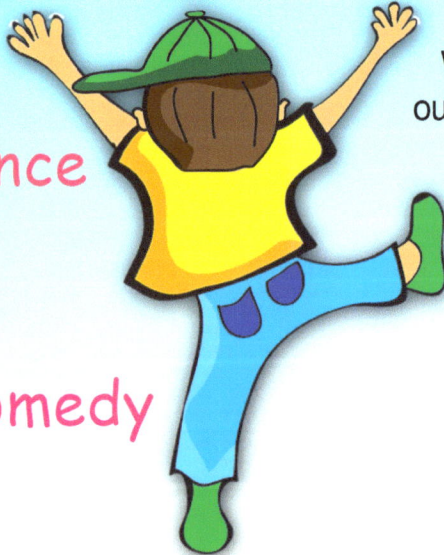

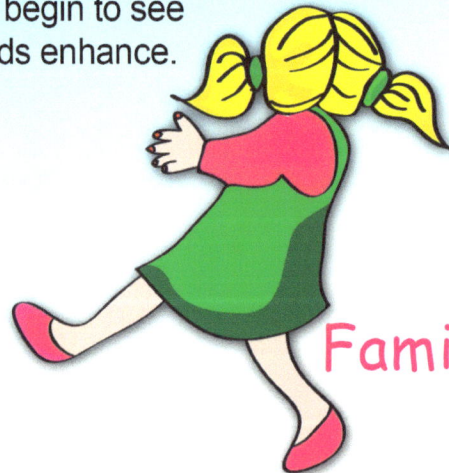

Comedy

Family Movies

COMPUTERS

Emails

News

Monitor Progress

Computers are
so useful at school.
They make learning
fun and cool.

They make our
thinking and reflexes fast.
Now spelling mistakes
are a thing of the past.

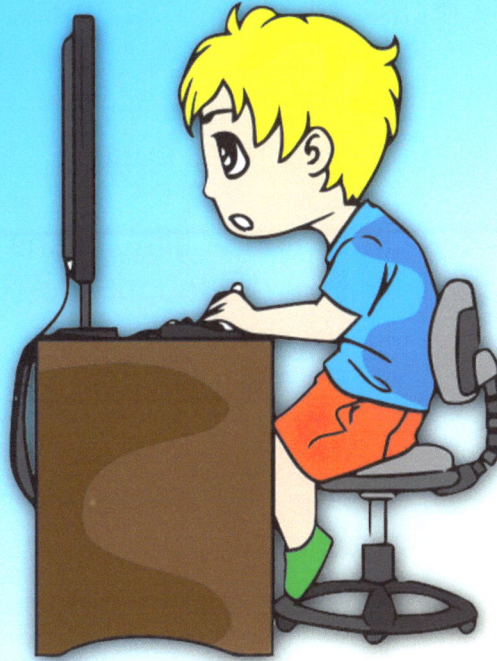

Within seconds,
we get connected
with the person
we intended.

Working becomes simple,
efficient, and fast.
It is much better
than working in the past.

Information

School Website

For every house and office,
they are now advisable.
Progressing without them
is now unthinkable.

Education

Books

**Better
Organization**

VIDEO GAMES

Fun

Games with family and friends
are so much fun
that we never ever
want to be done.

Puzzles

With computer simulations,
we are taught
many things while sitting
in a single spot.

Fast
Reflexes

Fitness
Games

Educational games
make us smarter
and teach us how to
think and act faster.

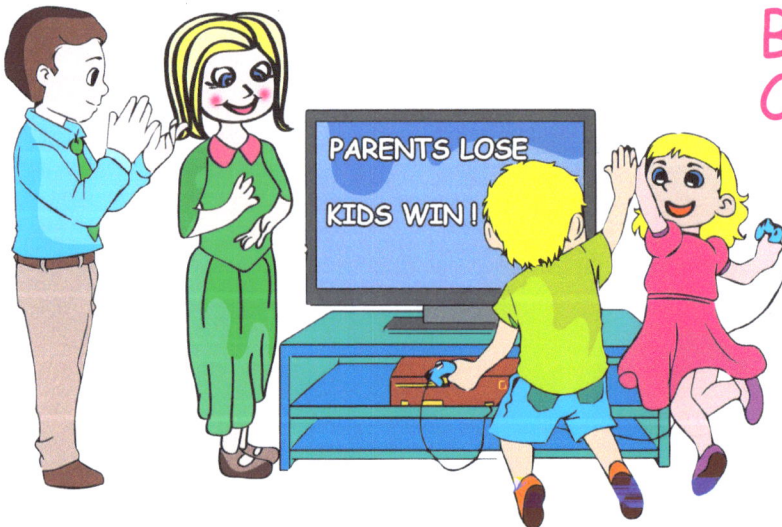

Better Hand Eye
Coordination

PARENTS LOSE

KIDS WIN !

AGGRESSIVE BEHAVIOR

POOR GRADES

OBESITY

DEPRESSION

NIGHTMARES

ADDICTION

POOR RELATIONSHIPS

BAD EFFECT ALERT !!!

The bad effects of the screen quietly sneak in. They live beside us and can harm us without our knowledge.

The biggest problem is that when we start watching television or playing video games, we find it very difficult to stop.

In video games, we either win, lose, or keep score. If we win, we want to win again and again. If we lose, we want to get better or improve our score. Therefore, we are not able to leave the screen: we are hooked!

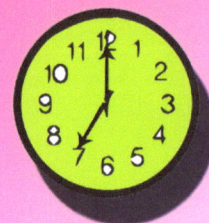

Dinner time!

Five more minutes?

Dinner time is family time.
Don't waste this precious time!

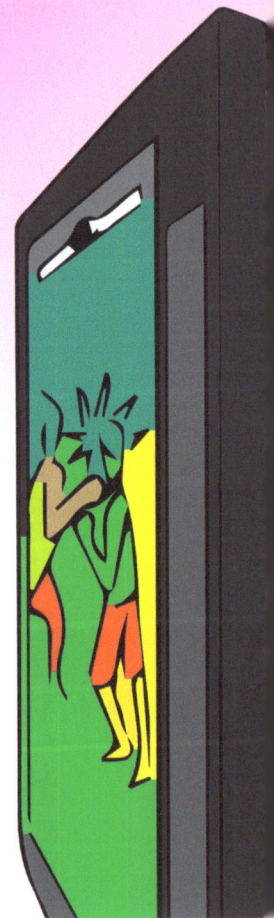

We miss our family time and forget to do fun activities like reading, coloring, doodling, and playing outside. We do not want to be told to turn off the screen. We begin to argue and fight with our family and friends.

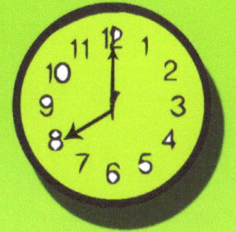

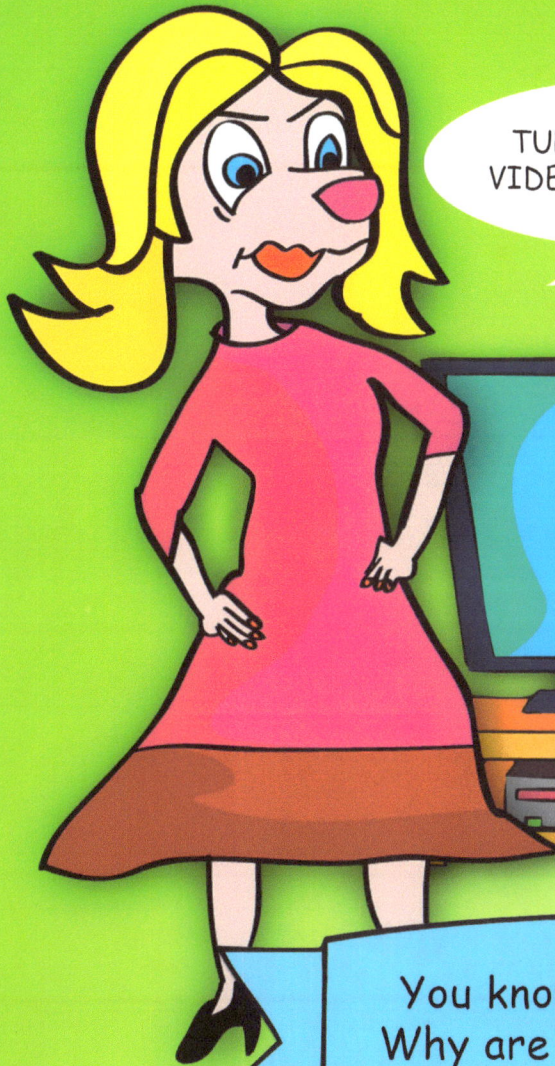

TURN OFF THIS VIDEO GAME NOW!

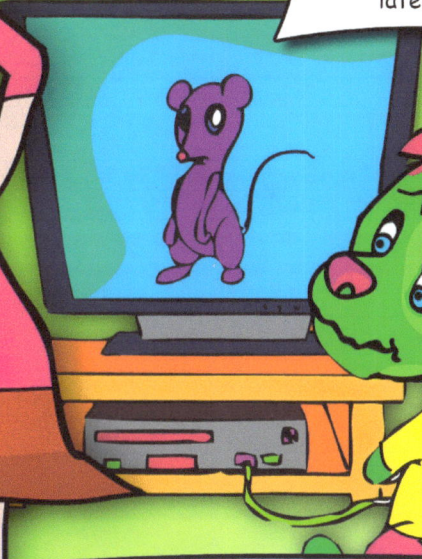

One hour later...

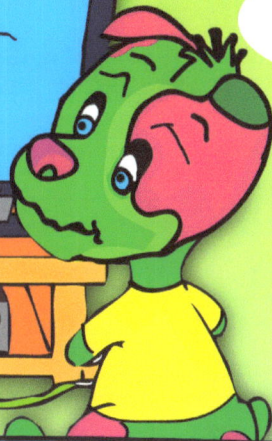

NO!!!

You know your mother is right. Why are you starting this fight?

When we are playing violent video games, we are actively participating in the fight scenes. When we watch or play these fight scenes again and again, we begin to feel that it is normal to fight to get whatever we want. We learn to become aggressive. Aggression could be simple like arguing over small things. Or it could be really bad like harming and hurting other people. We forget how to cooperate and work together as a team.

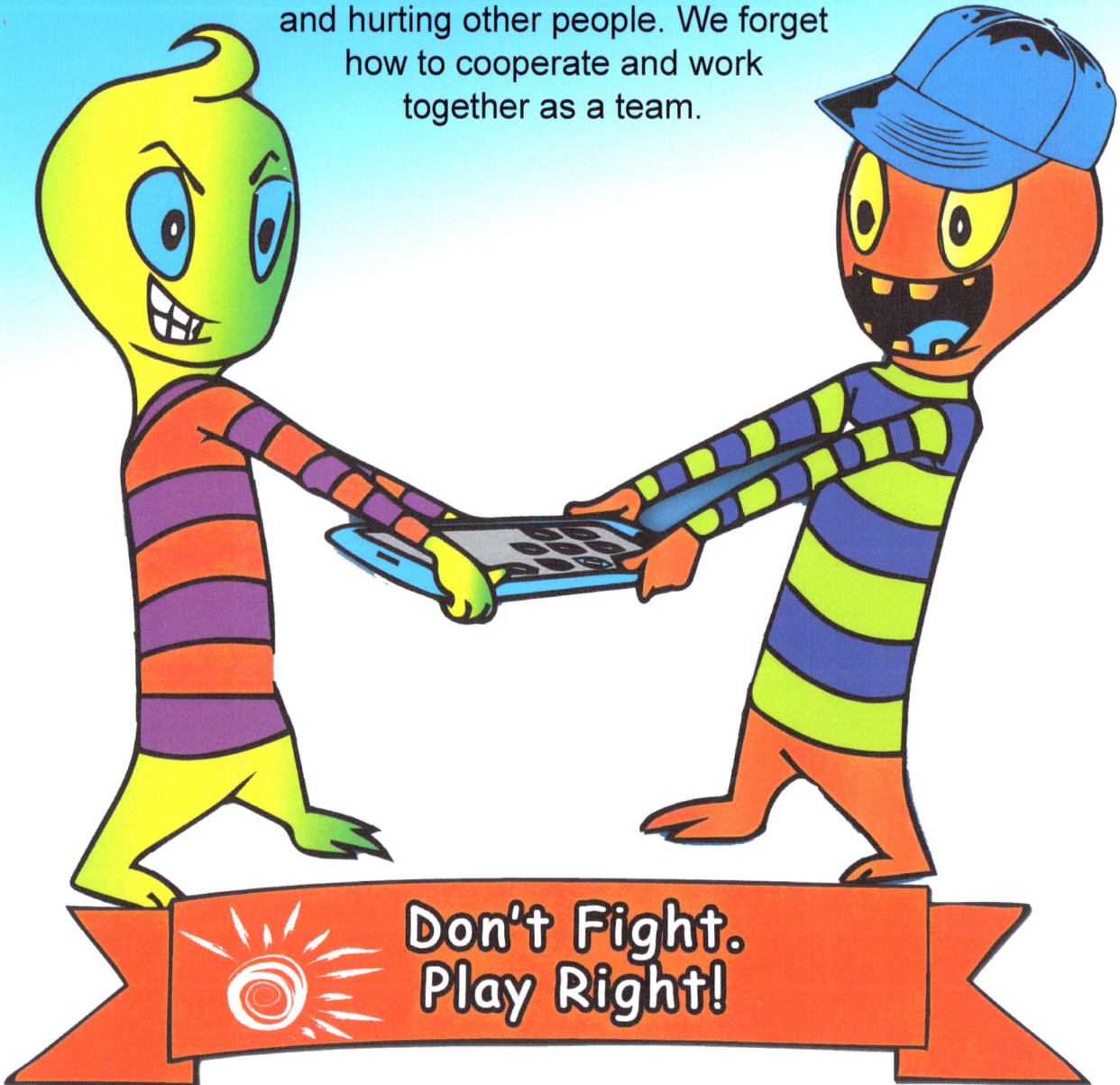

Don't Fight. Play Right!

Some television shows and certain
video games have scary scenes
in them. Too much involvement
with such games or programs
can scare us and make us feel
that the world is really bad.
We may not be able to
sleep well and may have
nightmares. This can
have a bad effect on
our development.

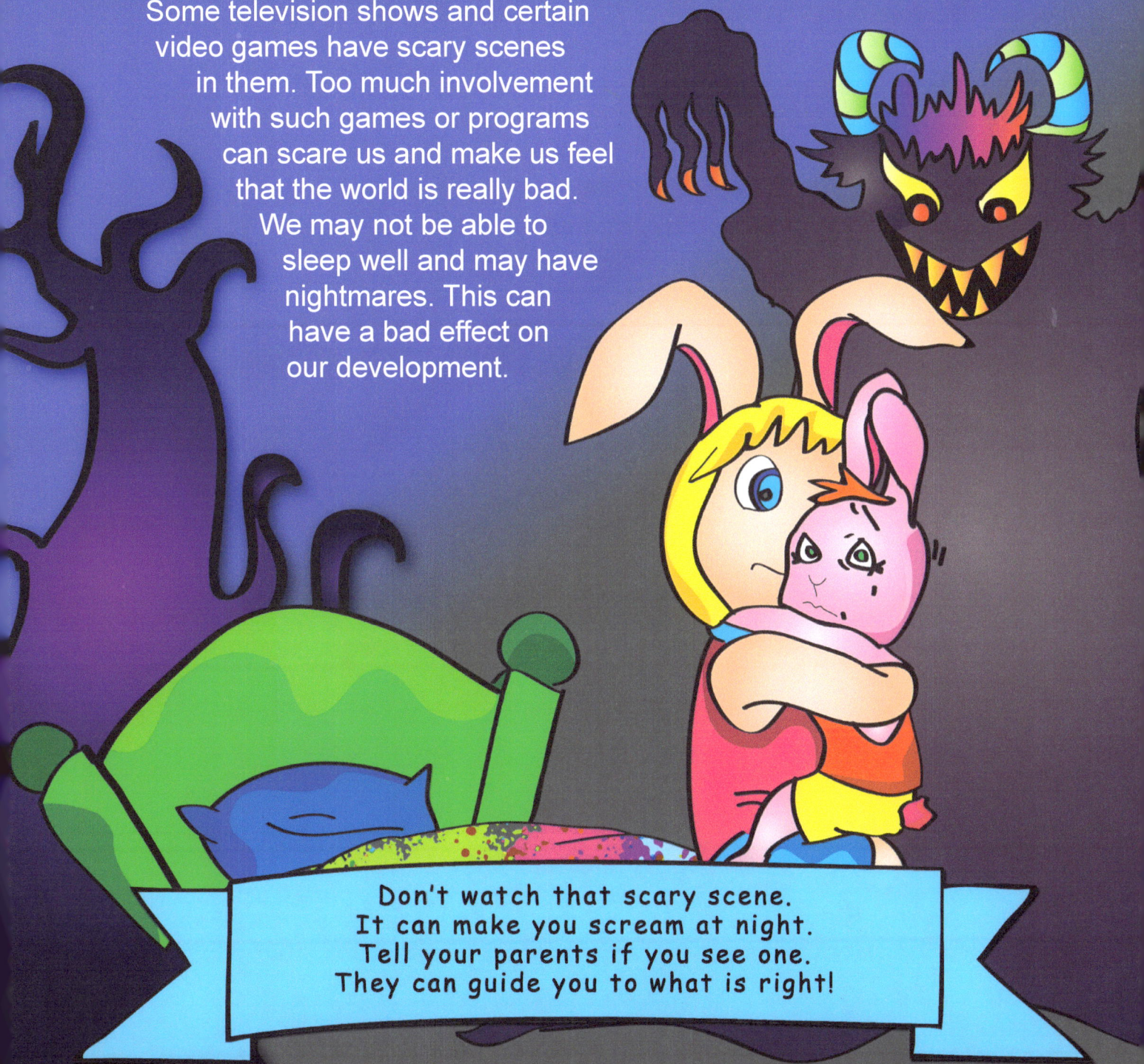

Don't watch that scary scene.
It can make you scream at night.
Tell your parents if you see one.
They can guide you to what is right!

If we are watching the screen for a long time, we get distracted and forget to do our homework. When we study and read on our own, our brain becomes stimulated. This makes us very smart. When we sit in front of the television, our brain doesn't think well, and it can make us dull. Therefore, we should not watch too much television or play video games for a very long time.

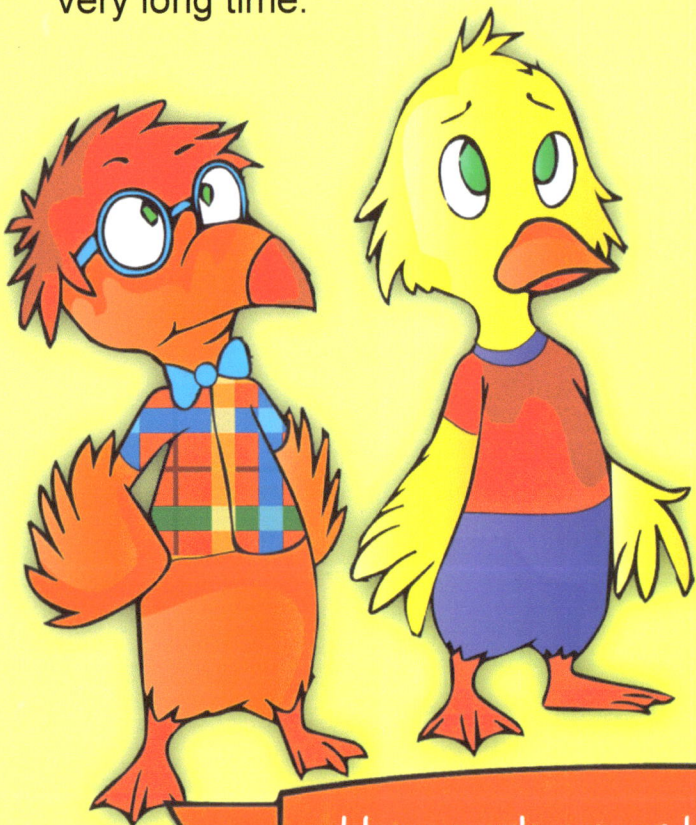

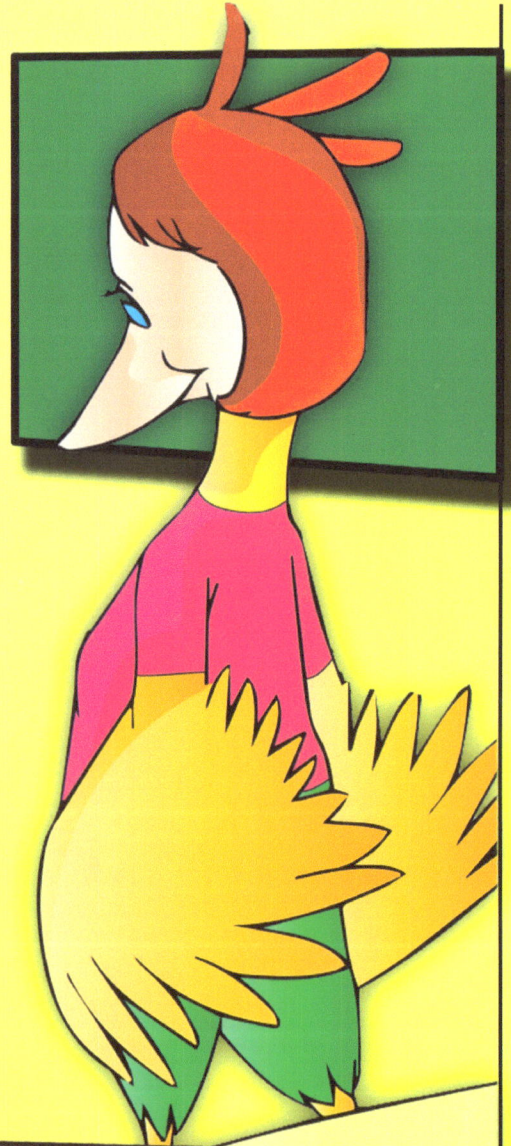

Homework comes before the screen.
This is what your teacher really means!

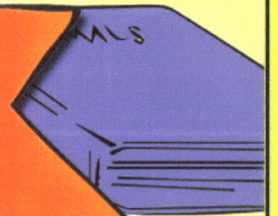

When we watch too much television or play too many video games, we often munch on snacks. Therefore, we tend to eat more than what is needed. Also, we do less physical activity. This can result in obesity and poor health habits. It can lead to diabetes and depression.

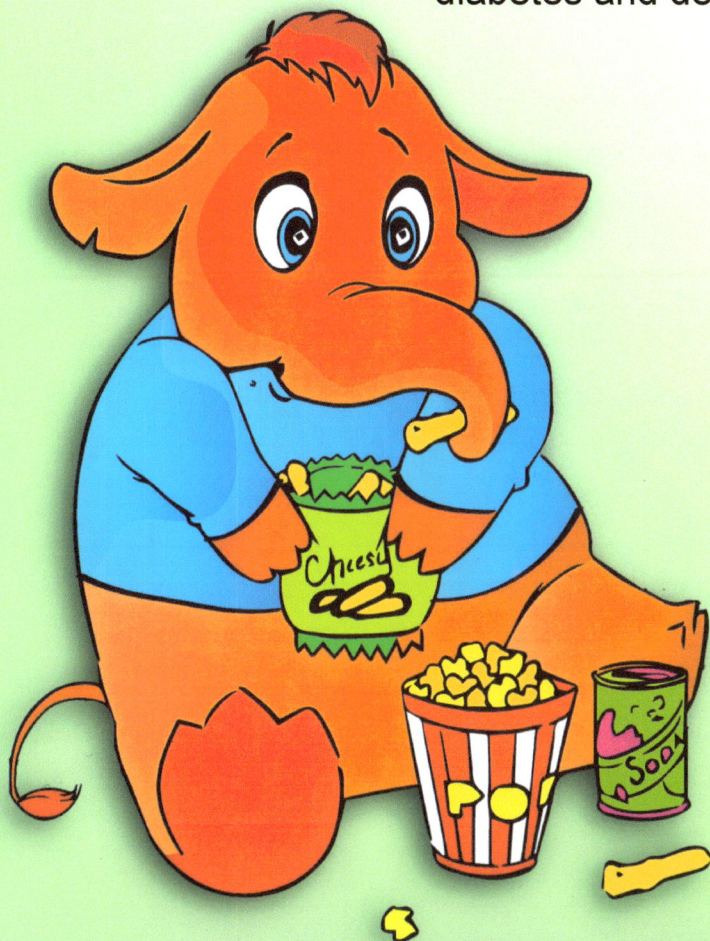

Don't overeat in front of the screen. It can definitely make you obese!

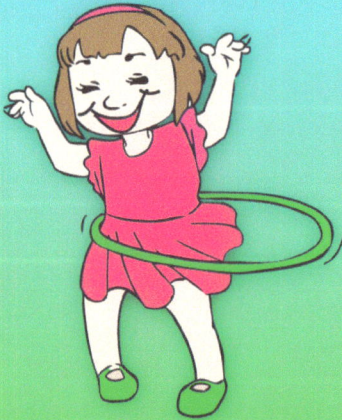

THIS IS WHAT THE DOCTORS RECOMMEND

We should not have a television, a computer, or a video game in our room. If we have one, then we tend to watch the screen for a longer time.

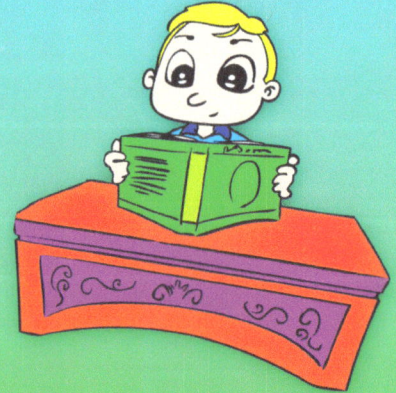

We should not watch the screen for more than two hours a day. This includes televisions, computers and video games.

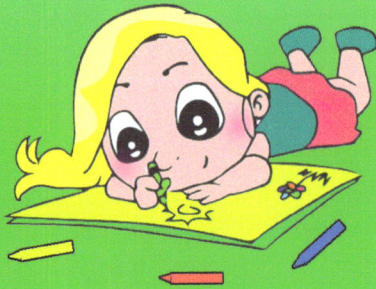

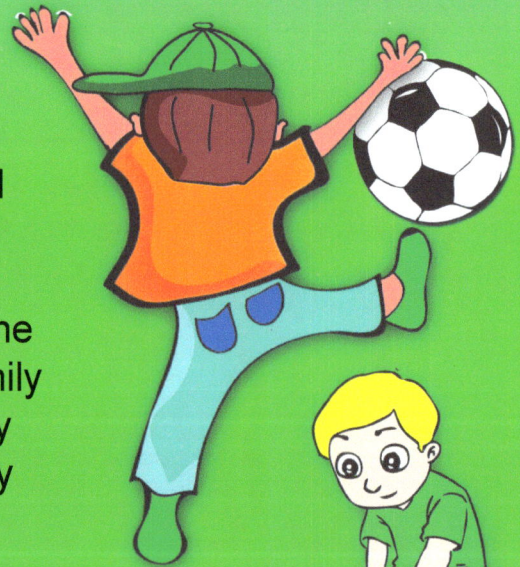

Screen time should be done as a group activity with family or friends. We should only watch good shows and play good games as recommended by our parents.

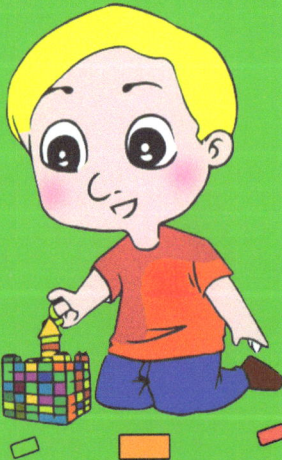

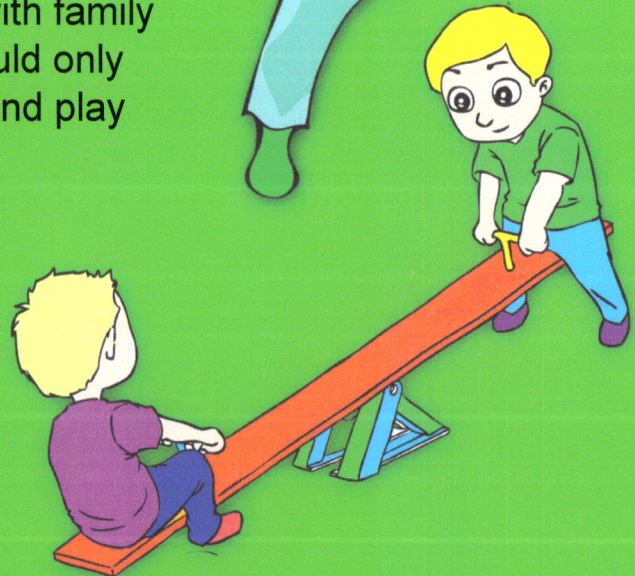

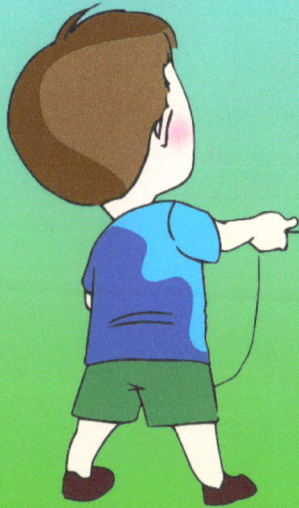

We should play outside and do other fun activities. Also, we should finish our homework before we start playing on the screen.

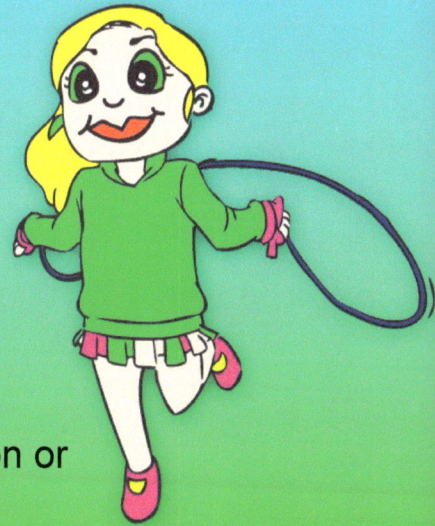

We should not let our siblings less than two years old watch any television or be on any device with a screen.

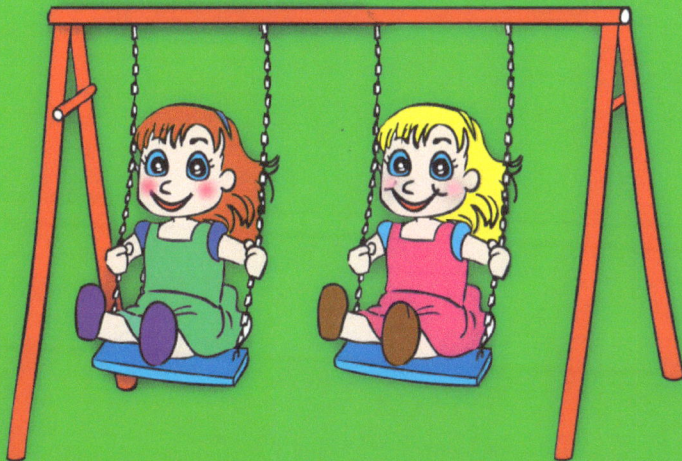

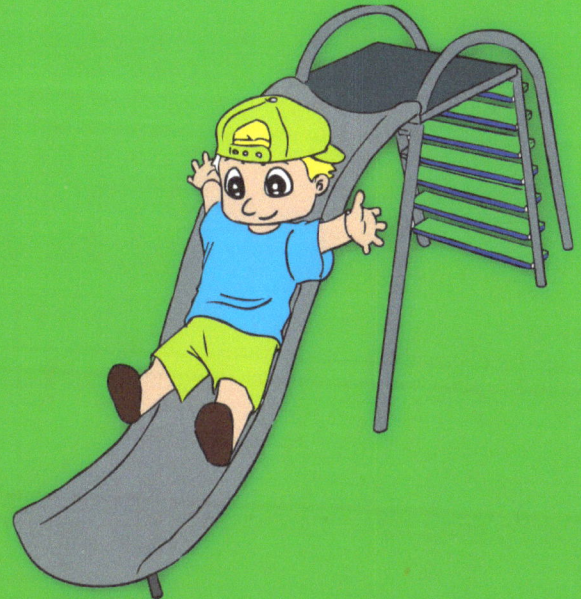

This is like a tug

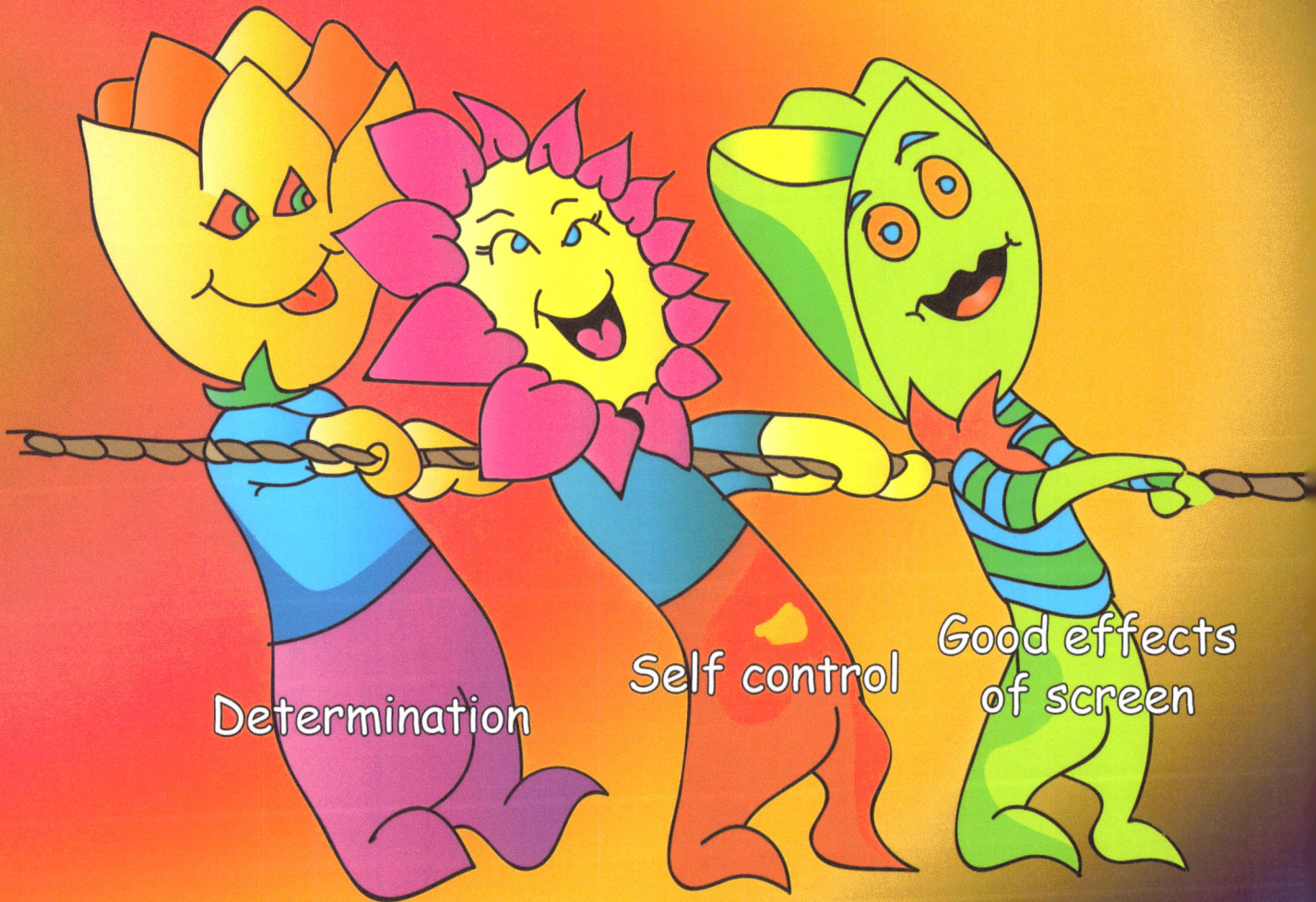

Determination

Self control

Good effects
of screen

Electronic devices have both positive and negative effects.

# of war between...

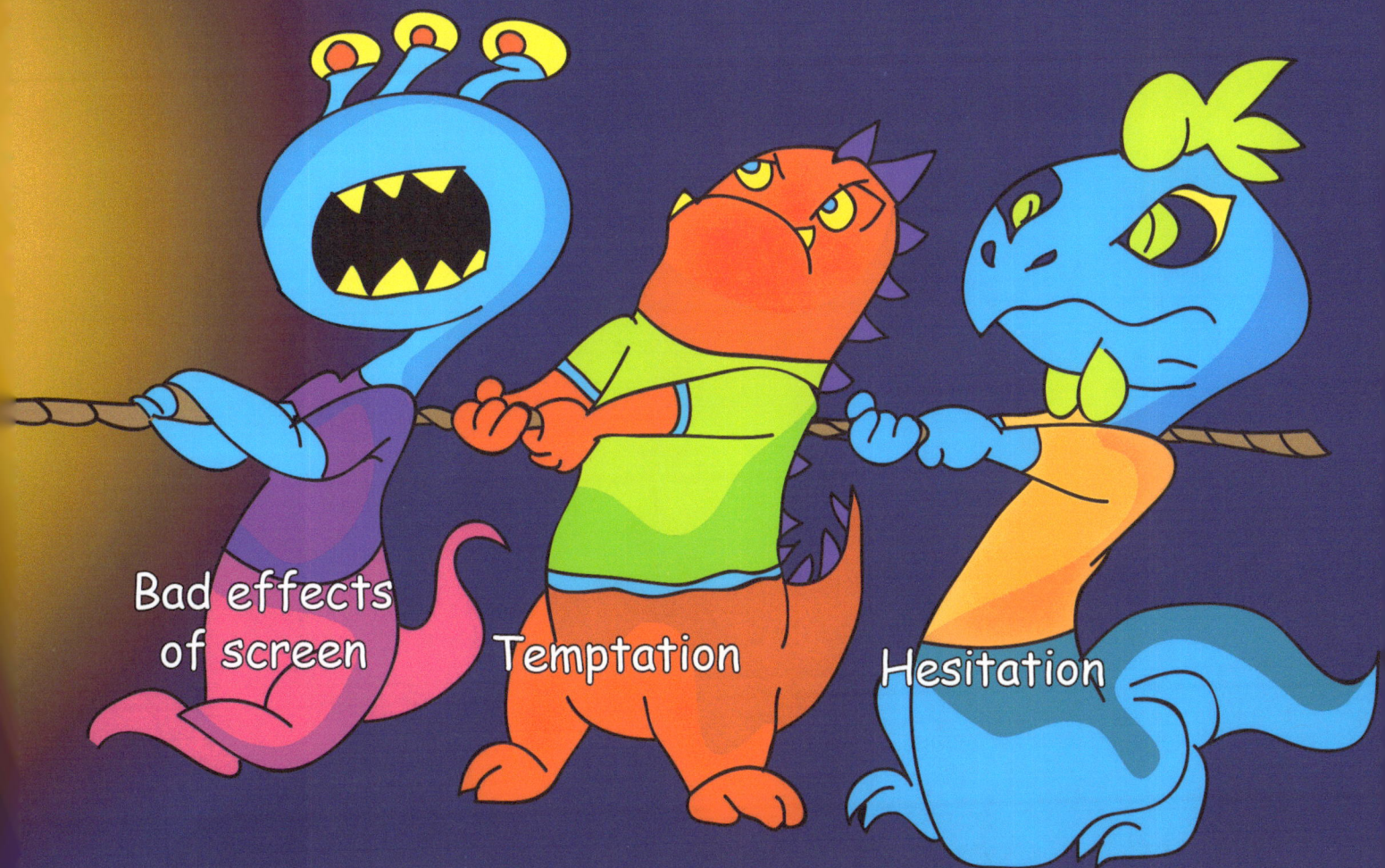

Bad effects
of screen

Temptation

Hesitation

Our self-control and determination can make the good side win.

Making the good side win is always in our hands.

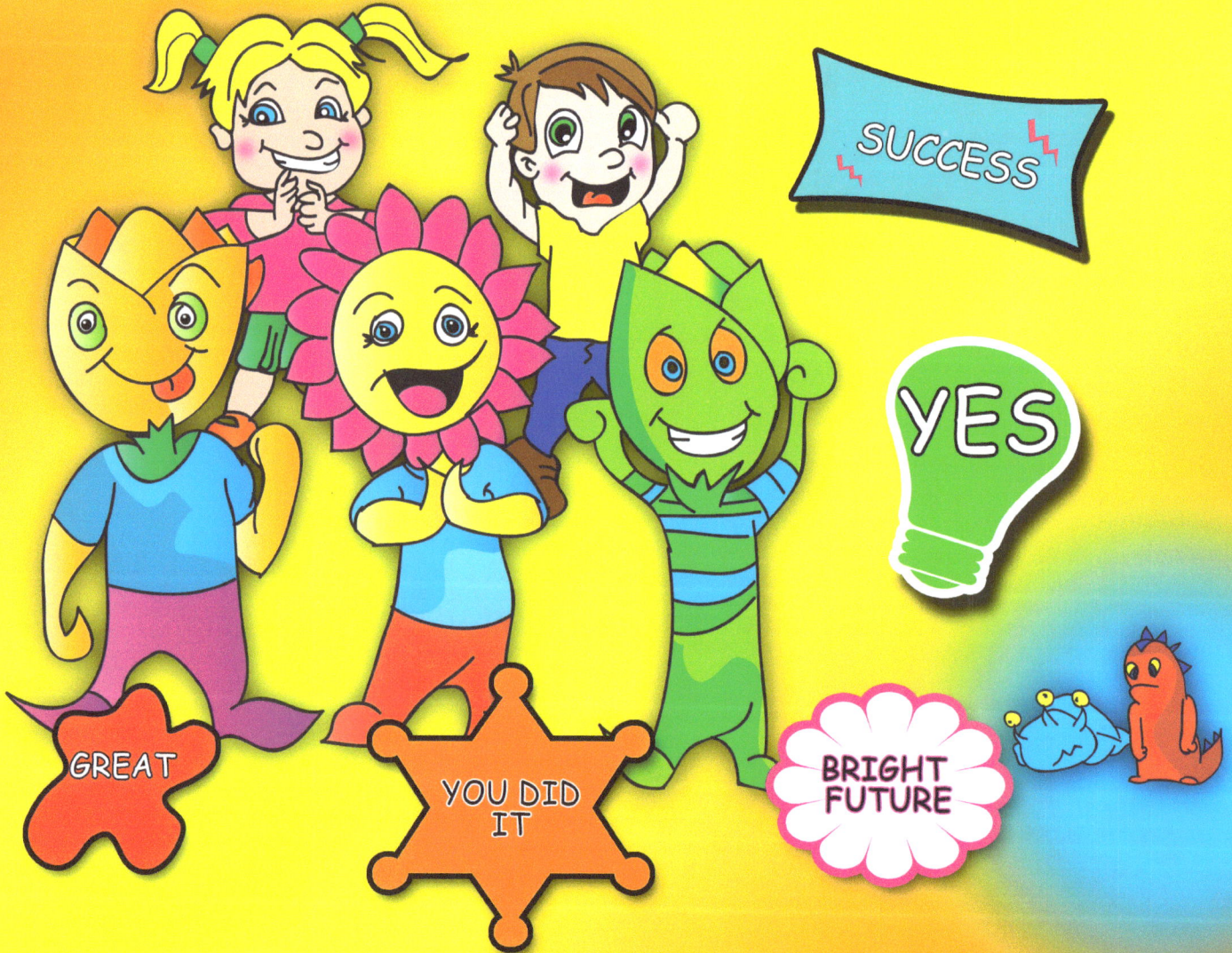

We watch television, play on computers and
video games,
but never more than two hours a day.
We always finish our homework first.
We read, play outside, and spend time with
our family and friends.

We are good children.
We are happy children.
Come join us!!!

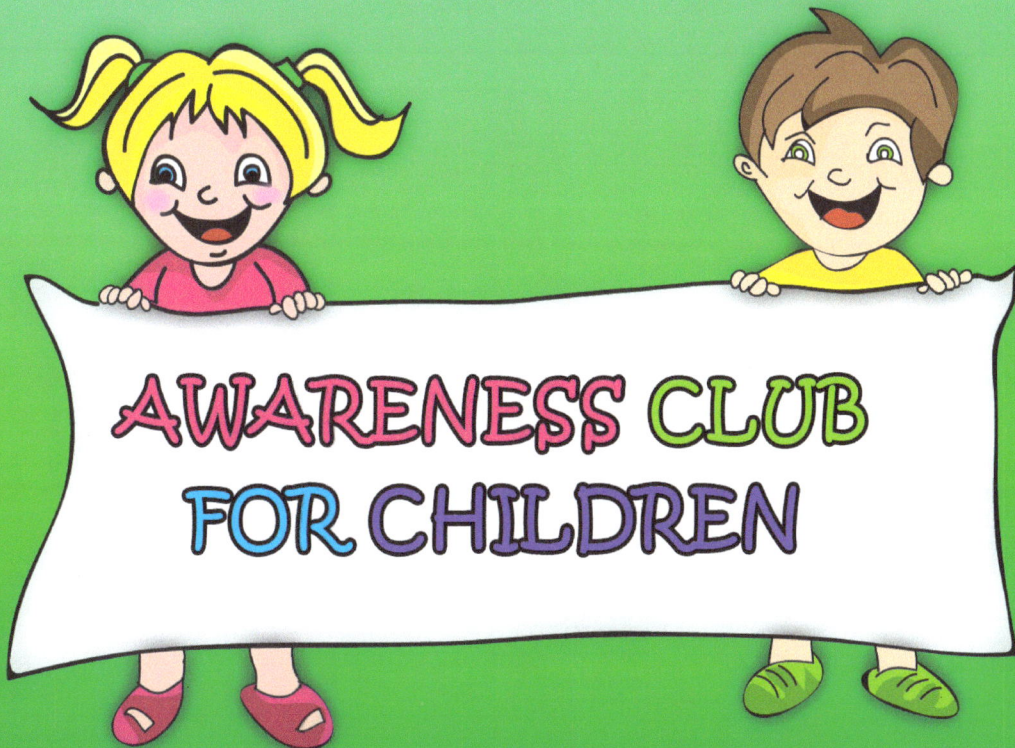

AWARENESS CLUB
FOR CHILDREN

Do things
on the screen
but control your time
is all we mean!

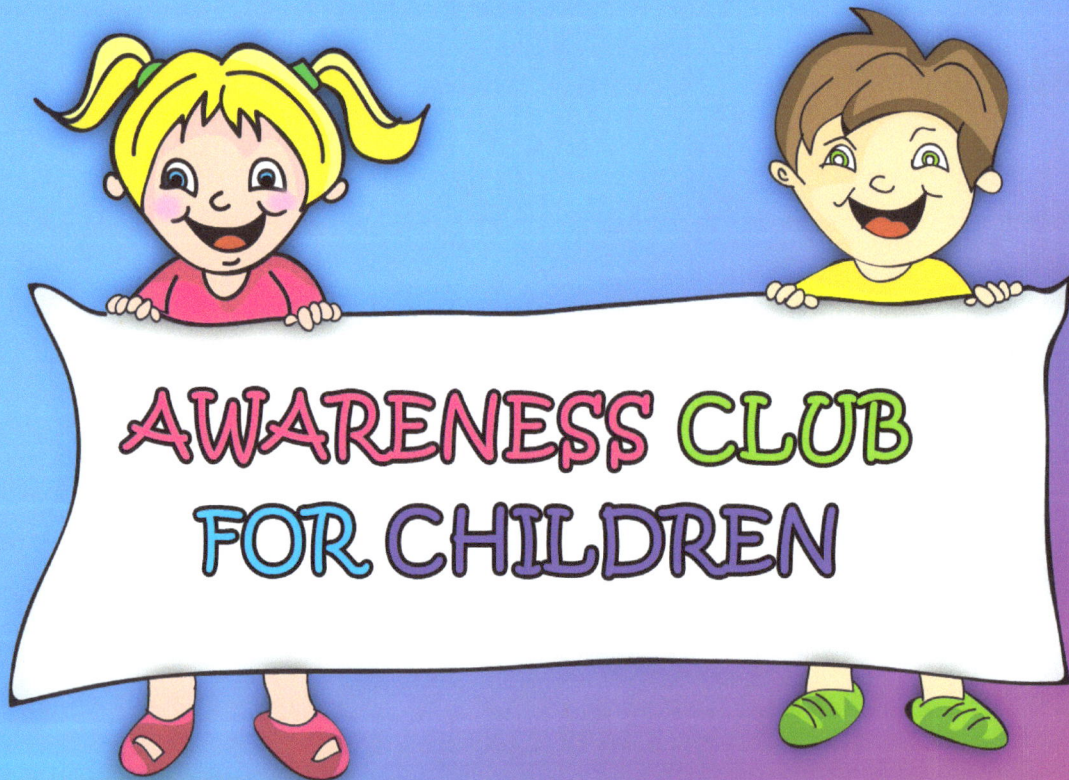

AWARENESS CLUB
FOR CHILDREN

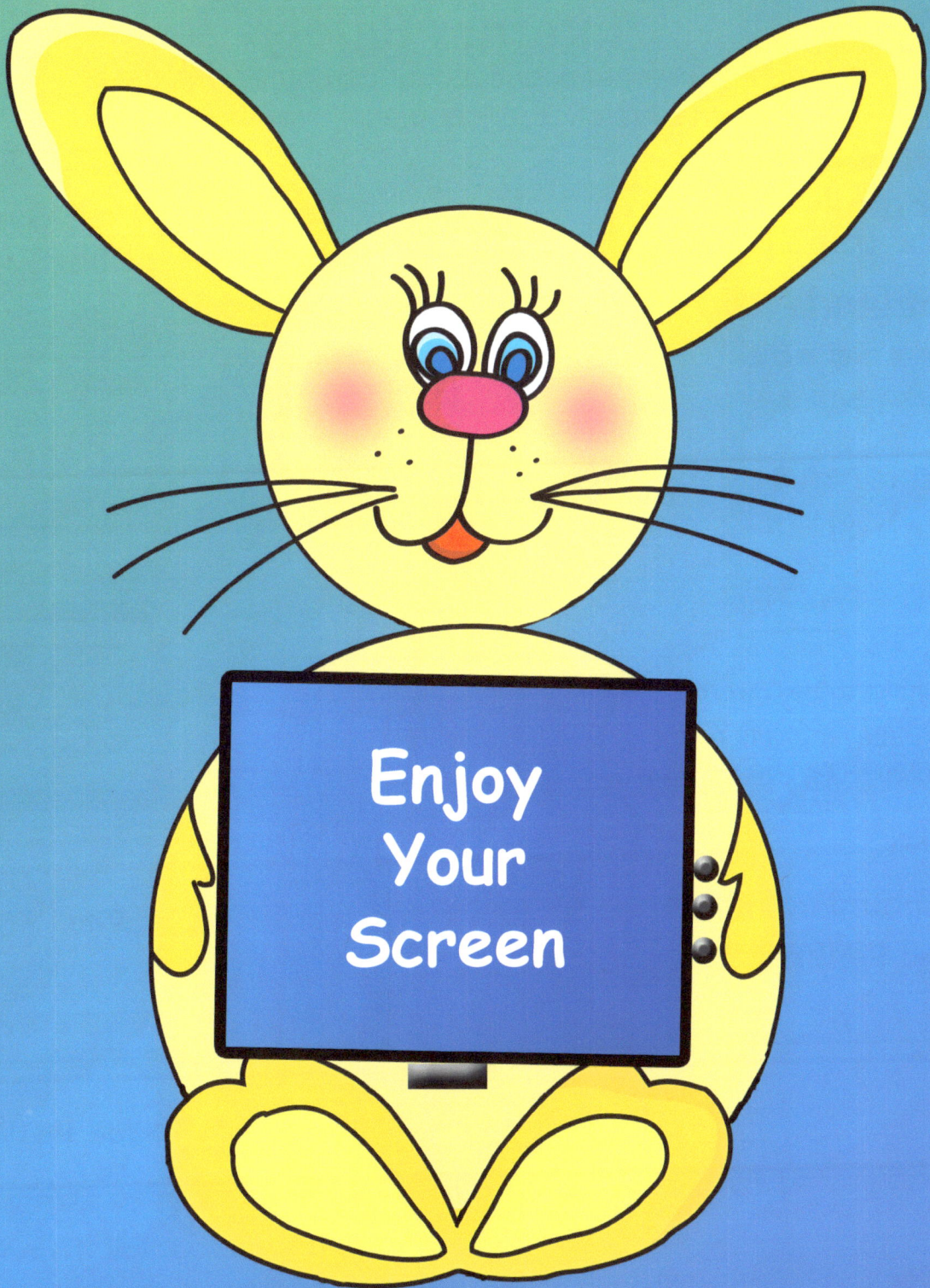
Enjoy Your Screen

Internet Safety

The Internet connects our computer with the computers of other people all over the world.

Family & Friends

Children's Web sites

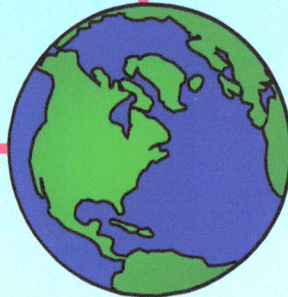

Free Game
Click Here

Search

Bunny

Enter your:
- **Name**
- **Date of Birth**
- **Address**

Copy   Paste

You are BAD!

I have to be **Careful!**
Whatever I write on the Internet can be seen by many people.

We should not share our password!

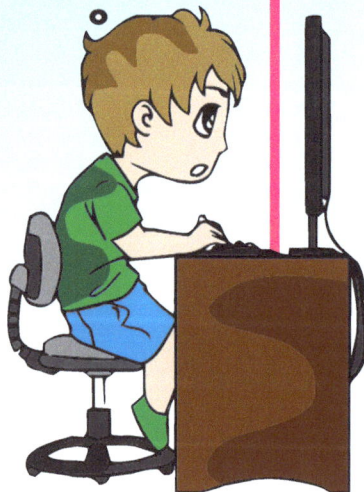

Clicking here is like opening the door of our house to a stranger. A person from anywhere in the world may be able to see the important information stored in our computer.

We should not download anything on our own.

When we type and search on our own, our computer can get connected to the people who can harm us. This is like going to a house of a stranger.

We should not search alone.

Bad people can use our information.

We should not give away our personal information

This is called plagiarism. We can be punished.

We should not copy and paste from the Internet.

This is bullying.

We should inform our teachers or parents.

The Internet is a crowded place with millions of computers.

Going on the Internet without an adult is like walking alone in a large, crowded city with lots of people. We can get lost and hurt.

We should never leave our house alone; similarly we should never go on the Internet alone.

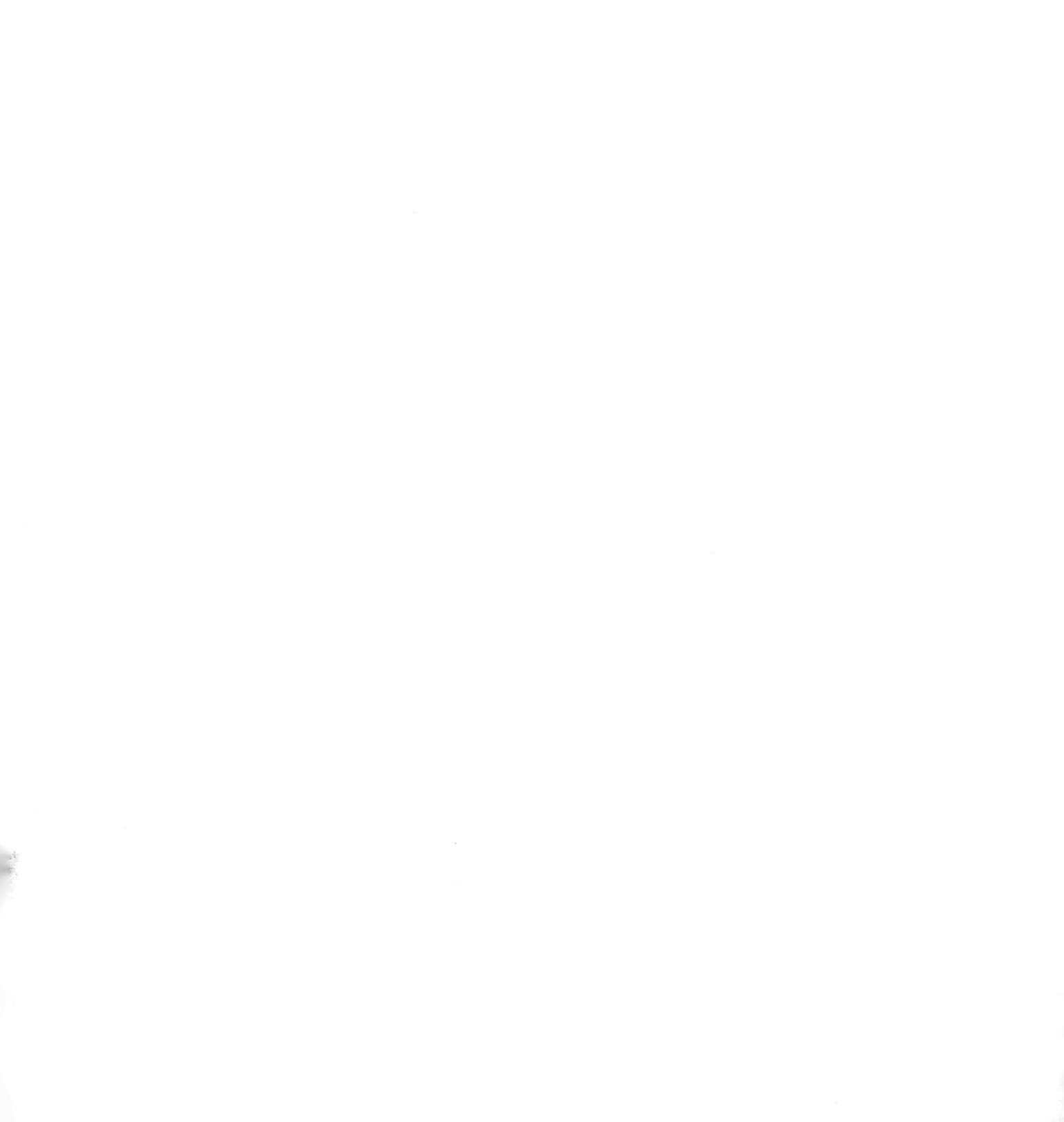

www.ingramcontent.com/pod-product-compliance
Lightning Source LLC
Chambersburg PA
CBHW041547260326
41914CB00016B/1575